Prevention:
The Most Important Treatment of Heart Disease

A Companion Guide: Using Diet and Exercise to Reduce Your Risk of a Heart Attack, Angioplasty, or Bypass Surgery

Gregg M. Yamada, M.D

Prevention: The Most Important Treatment of Heart Disease
Gregg M. Yamada, M.D.

Printed in the United States of America.

The Executive Diet, LLC
PO BOX 160901
Honolulu, HI 96816

ISBN-13: 978-1499697391
ISBN-10:1499697392

Cover design by Kelly Leslie
Book design by Christopher Fisher

This edition was prepared for printing by
The Editorial Department
7650 E. Broadway, #308, Tucson, Arizona 85710
www.editorialdepartment.com

*To my patients who encouraged me to share with others
what I share with them every day.*

Prevention: The Most Important Treatment of Heart Disease

Contents

Disclaimer

This book contains the opinions of its author and is not a medical manual. It is intended to be helpful and informational only. It is not a substitute for any advice or treatment prescribed by your own physician. Do not begin this or any other diet or exercise program, without the approval of your own personal physician. Consult with your personal physician prior to considering any of the suggestions in this book or drawing inferences from it.

The author expressly disclaims responsibility for any adverse effect which is incurred as a consequence of the use and application of the information contained in this book.

Mention of specific companies, organizations, or authorities in this book does not imply endorsement by the author or that they endorse this book.

Introduction

Before You Read This Book

Before you buy this book, I want to make sure that it's the right book for you. It may not be.

There are dozens of excellent books that have been written about cardiac prevention, diet, and exercise. This isn't intended to replace any of them. Rather, I'd like you to think of this book as a *companion guide* that reinforces what you already know about heart disease and are probably already doing regarding weight loss, diet, and exercise. *In fact, if you only have enough room for one prevention book on your shelf, this shouldn't be the one.* I recommend that you consider buying any of the excellent books written by leading cardiac experts from the Cleveland Clinic, the Mayo Clinic, Stanford University, or the Harvard Medical School. Those manuals are comprehensive and provide specific recommendations on lifestyle modification to help you prevent heart disease.

Although I associate with renowned heart specialists from leading medical institutions on a routine basis, I'm not one of them. I am simply a practicing cardiologist with many years of experience helping my patients—avoid having to see renowned heart specialists at leading medical institutions!

When it comes to preventing heart disease, I'm sure you are already familiar with the importance of lowering your cardiac risk factors, maintaining a healthy weight, following a diet low in cholesterol and saturated fat, and getting regular exercise. There's not much more I can add to that apart from reinforcing these important concepts.

Also, with regard to losing weight, this isn't a diet book in the traditional sense. In fact, I don't even have a diet program for you to follow. There are no original recipes or meal plans in this book. I also don't make any grandiose claims of how much weight you'll lose in two weeks, for example. Rather, I share some common-sense strategies to help you maintain your weight loss. Losing weight is obviously important, but it's *maintaining your weight loss* that is the overall goal.

I also don't have any exercise routines for you. Instead, I recommend that you take a 30-minute walk most days of the week.

So what's the purpose of a cardiac prevention book that repeats most of what you already know, has no original diet program, and whose exercise program only consists of walking a half-hour a day?

The problem is that in spite of all of the excellent

books about prevention, heart disease remains the number-one killer. Even with all of the available diet books and exercise videos the majority of Americans are overweight, and most don't exercise at all! Millions of people have poorly controlled high blood pressure, high cholesterol, and diabetes. Millions more still smoke! In other words, everyone knows what to do, so why aren't we doing a better job of preventing heart disease?

In order to answer this question, you'll need to completely change the way you think about prevention.

There are two key points that you should take away from this book. The first is to consider prevention to be an actual *treatment* of heart disease. Prevention is a treatment that you start ten to twenty years before you suffer a heart attack.

The second and most important message of this book is to *not give up* on your diet and exercise program. Persevere! Give your diet and exercise program another try. But this time, be a bit more patient with yourself. Cardiac prevention is a marathon, not a sprint. Adopting a healthy lifestyle isn't as easy as it sounds. In fact, it's extremely difficult. It takes patience to change a lifetime of diet and exercise habits.

We live in an impatient world and expect immediate and often unrealistic results. If you're impatient when it comes to losing weight or exercising, then you'll look for extreme solutions. Complicated diets or strenuous exercise programs are too difficult to follow. You'll quit and become frustrated. Allow yourself some room to make mistakes. Sure, there will be times when you didn't follow your diet as closely as you'd hoped to. You may not have been able to exercise as much as you would have liked or lost as much weight as you intended. You may have fallen short of your cholesterol goal. That's okay! Keep moving in the right direction—a little progress each day.

Here's a simple analogy. Think of your cardiac prevention program as if it were a summer road trip with your family. If you're driving across country, how do you plan your trip? Pack the kids in the car, fill up your gas tank, and drive as fast as you can? Of course not! You spend a lot of time planning a scenic and enjoyable route. You build flexibility into your schedule with enough time to explore different places along the way.

The point is that your family road trip, similar to adopting a healthy lifestyle, should be fun and enjoyable rather than a chore. Sure, there will be some ups and downs along the way, a flat tire, a lost hotel reservation, but that's expected. Those little setbacks won't cause you to turn your car around, will they? Of course not!

After You Read This

Schedule that follow-up visit with your doctor that you've been avoiding. It's okay that you didn't get around to following your doctor's instructions as closely as you should have. Sometimes life gets in the way! Talk it over with your doctor and hit the reset button. Create more realistic goals and timetables for losing weight, lowering your cholesterol, blood pressure, and blood sugar. Chances are that your doctor is just as impatient as you are! "Lose thirty pounds by the end of the year!" isn't prevention, and besides that, it's unrealistic.

Follow up with your primary care doctor every few months initially to make sure that your blood pressure, blood sugar, and cholesterol are improving. If you haven't met these goals but have made even a little progress, consider that to be a success! If your goal may have been to lose twenty pounds in six months, but you only lost five pounds, good work on losing those five pounds! Keep it up!

I wish you the very best success in staying healthy. *Remember, doing what you know is more important than knowing what to do.*

Gregg Yamada, M.D.

PART ONE:
PREVENTION

The Importance of Prevention: The Number-One Killer

Someone you know has heart disease. It could be one of your family members, a close friend, or a co-worker. It may even be you. Heart disease, or coronary artery disease, is the number-one killer of men and women. Combined with stroke, cardiovascular disease is responsible for more deaths than all forms of cancer, lung disease, and accidents—combined!

LEADING CAUSES OF DEATH
1. Heart Disease and Stroke (cardiovascular disease)
2. Cancer
3. Lung Disease
4. Accidents

Source: Murphy, SL, et al.: National Vital Statistics Reports. 2013;61(4)

In the United States, someone suffers a heart attack every thirty seconds, and someone dies from one every sixty seconds. Tragically, most people who experience a myocardial infarction die before their ambulance reaches the hospital. Even if you are fortunate enough to make it to the hospital your chances are only one in four of surviving to your next birthday. These are sobering statistics, and you need to avoid being one of them.

Emergency room doctors have a saying: "Everyone eventually passes through the E.R." Many people also believe that heart disease is "inevitable" and "just happens." I disagree. Having a heart attack is not a foregone conclusion. Angioplasty or bypass surgery is not your destiny. There isn't a cardiac stent with your name on it.

HEART DISEASE IN WOMEN

1. Leading cause of death of women

2. A woman dies from heart disease every minute.

3. 1 in 3 deaths in women is due to heart disease, more than all forms of cancer combined.

4. 1 in 31 American women die of breast cancer vs. 1 in 3 women who die from heart disease.

5. Only 1 in 5 women think that heart disease is their biggest health risk

Source: Roger V, et.al. *Circulation*. 2013;127:e6-e245

You need to stay healthy and avoid the emergency room. Staying healthy *is* prevention. If you give your best effort to making the necessary lifestyle changes to avoid heart disease and cancer, chances are good you'll live to a very old age.

When it comes to your heart health there are three events you *can* prevent:

A heart attack

An angioplasty or stent

A bypass surgery

If you've already suffered a heart attack or had an angioplasty or a bypass surgery, there are three events you *must* prevent:

A second heart attack

A second angioplasty or stent

A second bypass surgery

No, we can't prevent all heart disease. But you can certainly do a great deal to avoid becoming a cardiology statistic. In addition to the obvious dangers of heart disease, there's also the added cost and inconvenience. Think of all the time you'll waste just in your doctor's waiting room alone! Then there's the expense of endless doctor appointments, tests, procedures, and medications. You need to do all you can to avoid this.

Now for the good news. Did you know that you can reduce your chance of suffering or dying of a heart attack by 30-40% just by walking thirty minutes a day? Seems really easy, doesn't it? Yet, most people don't make time to perform any exercise at all. We're just too busy.

Please don't misconstrue my message. I don't want you to avoid doctors or hospitals if you have a medical problem. If you have heart disease, you need to be under a cardiologist's care. But if you do all that you can to prevent heart disease, you may not ever *need* a cardiologist.

About This Book

I've divided this book into two sections. The first section is about a preventive approach to heart health. The second half covers weight loss, diet, and exercise.

Because your primary care physician is already managing your blood pressure, cholesterol, and blood sugar and has educated you on the importance of lowering these risk factors, I'll only briefly cover these issues. You may be tempted to skip right to the section on diet, but resist the urge. Skim through the pages about cardiac risk factors if you want, but try to spend some time understanding my approach to prevention. You have to really buy into the concept that prevention is a *treatment* of heart disease. If you don't agree with this, you'll have little motivation to change your lifestyle. Without this necessary background information, my recommendations for diet and exercise won't be as effective.

The emphasis in the second part of this book is on *maintaining* the weight reduction you achieve through dieting. Once you choose a diet plan that you feel comfortable following, I'll explain two strategies which will help you keep the weight off.

1. *Knowing how much to eat each day*—your calorie equilibrium.

2. *Curbing your appetite and junk food cravings*—no diet will work if you're always hungry all the time.

A Different Type of Prevention Book: A Companion Guide

This is a book about prevention, although you'll find it to be a lot different from others you may have read. It's really more of a *companion guide* to more comprehensive prevention books. My goal is to help you reduce your risk of heart disease through simple lifestyle changes. I'll share some common-sense strategies to help you lose weight and, more importantly, keep it off.

But remember, preventing heart disease requires more than just losing weight, eating healthy, and exercising regularly. You'll need to reduce *all* your risk factors—including your weight. The modifiable cardiac risk factors for heart disease, as you already know, are hypertension, diabetes, hypercholesterolemia, smoking, and obesity. Weight loss is just one part of your *overall* preventive approach to heart disease. Modifying your diet and increasing your exercise are steps *you can take* to prevent heart disease. Controlling your hypertension, diabetes, and hypercholesterolemia are steps that *your doctor can help you take.*

Finally, there is no role for prevention in an emergency. You can't diet your way out of an angioplasty, and you can't exercise your way out of a bypass surgery. Weight loss doesn't help during a heart attack. Prevention is something you do ten years before a heart attack, bypass surgery, or angioplasty.

A Different Type of Diet Plan: Weight Maintenance versus Weight Loss

If you're overweight—and most Americans are—losing that excess weight is the most important step you can take to prevent heart disease. For one thing, weight loss improves your blood pressure, blood sugar, and cholesterol. Also, losing weight makes it easier for your doctor to lower your other risk factors. It may at least make it possible for you to decrease your medications, or perhaps even discontinue them *with your physician's approval.*

Unfortunately, you will have to be disciplined and follow a diet and exercise plan in order to lose weight. I don't have a specific diet plan for you to follow, because my focus is to help you keep the weight off rather than helping you lose weight. Let me explain.

Diets help you lose weight but don't necessarily help you keep from regaining it. Despite all the benefits of losing weight in preventing heart disease, there's absolutely no benefit if you gain it all back. Since there are already dozens of excellent diets for you to choose from, I didn't see the benefit of creating another diet.

Rather, I focused on developing simple strategies to help you maintain your healthier weight.

So find a diet that fits your lifestyle and get started!

What This Book Is Not

This is not a medical manual. You'll find very few references to medical journals, because this isn't a text-book either. By presenting a fresh perspective on how we *should* approach heart disease, I hope to motivate you to continue living a healthy lifestyle.

You already know what you have to do and why you have to do it. If you have high blood pressure, lower it. If your cholesterol is too high, then eat properly and lower this too. If you are overweight, eat less and start exercising regularly. If you smoke you know what to do!

Naturopathic or Holistic Medicine

Although I hope you can reduce your dependency upon medications through weight loss, diet, and exercise, I am not "anti-medication." If you're looking for holistic alternatives to prescription medications, this book is not for you. My knowledge of naturopathic or holistic medicine is limited at best. Rather, I am a cardiologist who follows standard-of-care medical guidelines to prevent heart disease.

Of course, I would rather you not take medications, if diet and exercise allow you to do without them, but this may not be possible. Getting off medications is not your primary goal. It is a secondary goal. Your primary goal should be achieving target values for blood pressure, blood sugar, and cholesterol by any means possible—with or without medications, under your doctor's supervision.

Prevention Is Never a Substitute for Proper Medical Care

Over the past forty years we've made tremendous advances in treating and preventing heart disease. Heart surgery and angioplasty techniques coupled with pharmaceutical breakthroughs not only save lives, they also improve the quality of life.

But remember, prevention is *never* a substitute for cardiac medications, bypass surgery, or angioplasty. If you have heart disease and your cardiologist recommends medications, tests, and procedures, please follow your doctor's advice. Don't make the mistake of thinking you can treat heart disease with weight loss, diet, and exercise. That could be a potentially fatal mistake on your part. If your doctor recommends angioplasty or bypass surgery and you're not comfortable with his recommendations, then get a second opinion from the most experienced cardiologist or cardiac surgeon at your local hospital and have your procedure performed as soon as possible. If you're not satisfied with local physicians and you doctor feels it is safe to do so, refer yourself to a leading cardiac hospital.

As I have said before, there is no role for prevention

in a heart attack, just as there is no role for prevention if you need bypass surgery or angioplasty. The time to think about preventing heart disease is ten *years* before you suffer a heart attack or require a stent or bypass surgery, not ten *days* before.

After you recover from your heart procedure, *then* you can adopt principles of cardiac prevention. "Primary prevention" refers to measures you take prior to a cardiac event (bypass, angioplasty, or heart attack) whereas "secondary prevention" is what you do to prevent a second one.

Prevention Is Not a Substitute for Your Own Doctor's Advice

I am a doctor, but I'm not your doctor. This book is not a substitute for your doctor's advice. *Never* change or stop medications without the approval of your personal physician. Never begin any new diet or exercise program without first consulting your doctor to be sure that it is safe for you.

Can Heart Disease Be Prevented?

Heart disease can be prevented. I believe this. Just about everybody believes this intuitively. Heart disease is preventable because we know what the causes are. By simply *lowering your cholesterol, controlling your blood pressure and blood sugar, losing weight, performing regular exercise, and stopping smoking,* you can dramatically reduce your chances of suffering a heart attack or needing bypass surgery or angioplasty. This is common knowledge and common sense.

Why Don't We Do a Better Job at Preventing Heart Disease?

So if it's that simple to prevent heart disease and we all know what to do, why aren't we doing it? Why is heart disease still the number-one killer of adults despite all the life-saving advances made in the past forty years?

There are several reasons for this.

Heart Disease Is Increasing, Not Decreasing

For one thing, the number of people with heart disease is overwhelming and ever-increasing. The statistics are staggering. In the United States alone, more than two thousand people die *each day* from complications of heart disease and stroke. A third of these people are under the age of 65. This is why the number of cardiac procedures increases each year, when we'd hope it would decrease. This year alone, more than one million angioplasties and more than four hundred thousand bypass surgeries will be performed in the U.S. At a time when we're in the midst of drastic changes in our healthcare system in order to lower costs of medical care, the total cost of *treating* heart disease this year will exceed 450 billion dollars. Heart disease is not only the most lethal disease, it is also the most expensive.

Procedure-Oriented Medical System

With heart disease so rampant and so costly, our entire medical system has been forced to focus upon treating heart disease rather than preventing it. Cardiologists and cardiac surgeons are so busy performing angioplasties and bypass surgeries that we don't have time to emphasize prevention. In current terms, treatment of heart disease typically refers to *angioplasty* or *bypass surgery*. The result is that our entire healthcare system is procedure-oriented. This circumstance influences how cardiologists are trained and how insurance carriers reimburse physicians and hospitals.

Fortunately, in the past forty years tremendous advances have taken place in angioplasty and bypass surgery. But this progress has required cardiologists and surgeons to become increasingly specialized, requiring even more years of training and additional board certifications. This is only logical, because professional medical societies must ensure that a physician has received the proper training and is competent to perform the latest procedures.

But with each passing year cardiology training becomes increasingly biased towards new treatment approaches, with less emphasis upon prevention. Consider the following career path choices. Following medical school, a typical cardiologist completes six years of training: three years of internal medicine, three years of general cardiology. Following two board certifications in internal medicine and general cardiology, the subsequent choices are to remain a general cardiologist or pursue specialized training in areas such as interventional cardiology (angioplasty) or electrophysiology (disturbances of heart rhythm). These require one or two additional years of training with another board certification. My own background included training and board certifications in internal medicine, general cardiology, interventional cardiology, nuclear cardiology, and cardiac CT imaging.

The point is this. Despite all the training that I have received and all the board-certifying examinations I have taken, there were no lectures and only a handful of exam questions dealing with prevention. Our focus is on the treatment of heart disease rather than prevention.

Don't get me wrong, as cardiologists we *want* to prevent heart disease. It's just not our priority at three o'clock in the morning when we're performing your emergency angioplasty.

Financial and Professional Reward

You may not know that our system rewards, both economically and professionally, those doctors and hospitals responsible for the highest number of procedures.

For example, a heart surgeon who performs three hundred surgeries per year will bring in more revenue to the hospital, earn the highest salary, and enjoy the professional stature of being "the best." This is reasonable, because you certainly don't want your bypass operation performed by a surgeon who performs very few such procedures. Also, the doctor who has more training and is performing a larger number of procedures should be paid more than one who is less specialized or has a low surgical load.

But the fact remains that the entire hospital staff, from the board of directors to the CEO right down to the nursing staff, knows who the high-volume operators are. Vendors of cardiac stents and surgical supplies to the hospital cater to doctors who perform a large number of procedures. There is nothing wrong with any of this, but it may help you understand how our system has evolved.

On the other hand, there is little or no recognition for your primary care doctor who performs no procedures but can help you avoid a bypass surgery. Our system doesn't reward prevention, it rewards treatment.

Insurance Carriers Don't Cover Preventive Testing

Most people aren't aware that Medicare and private insurance companies do not allow you to have preventive cardiac testing. Insurance carriers will pay for your bypass surgery bill, which may exceed three hundred thousand dollars, but they won't pay for a preventive test costing a few hundred dollars that can help you avoid your bypass.

Here's an example. Are you familiar with a heart scan or calcium score? If your blood vessels contain cholesterol deposits, over time those deposits become calcified. For more than twenty years doctors have known that the most accurate way to determine whether you have heart disease is by a calcium score. A CT scanner using low-dose radiation is able to detect calcium build-up in cholesterol plaques within your coronary arteries. Tabulation of this amount of calcium is known as a calcium score. The higher your score, the more likely you are to have a heart attack over the next five years. Naturally, you'll want the lowest score possible.

Based on this simple calcium score, we can get an idea of your future risk of a heart attack, whether you need further testing, what type of testing, and whether you need to begin taking a statin to lower your cholesterol. This single test, a cardiologist's most important tool, only costs about three hundred dollars, but medical insurance won't cover it because it is considered preventive. Most people don't realize that private insurance and Medicare consider preventive tests unnecessary!

Prevention on the Back Burner

But I've touched before on the most important reason why we aren't doing a better job of preventing heart disease: It's simply that we don't make prevention a priority in our daily lives.

Why is that? For one thing, no one wants to think about having a heart attack or a bypass surgery. No one wants to think about being sick. I certainly don't. You don't either. It's depressing. We all want to be healthy. It's a fact, nevertheless, that if you want to avoid heart disease, you must consider your risk factors and the consequences of not lowering them.

Another reason why prevention is put on the back burner is because everyone's busy. It takes a lot of time to watch what you eat and work out regularly. You know you should do these things, but it's difficult to find—or make—the time. When was the last time you told your doctor, "I'm too busy to exercise now," or "I can't stop smoking now because I'm under a lot of stress," or "I'd like to lower my cholesterol, but I have a cruise in a few months to Europe, and I know my cholesterol will be high."

Preventing heart disease by lowering our risk factors must be top of mind, not just a once-a-year lecture from your doctor.

Can We Prevent All Heart Disease?

I wish this were the case, but unfortunately not all heart disease can be prevented. There are two reasons why this is so.

First, the risk factors of age and family history are obviously not under our control.

Another difficulty is that coronary artery disease is usually "silent" and develops over many years with no warning. It's difficult to prevent a condition that you don't know you have. Most people who suffer a heart attack have little or no warning symptoms. In fact, the first time your doctor even knows you have heart disease is often when you suffer your first heart attack! Unfortunately, the outcome of a heart attack is typically death.

You can't change your age or genetics, but you can still do something to reduce your chances of a heart attack. Let me explain. If your mother or father suffered a heart attack at age 50, then you have a greater risk for heart disease. That is known as family history.

But even though you can't change who your parents

are, is there anything that you can do? Of course there is! Remember, the risk factors for heart disease are hypertension, diabetes, hypercholesterolemia, smoking, family history, obesity, and sedentary lifestyle, among other things. Simply reduce your other risk factors. This is the same advice that I give patients when they tell me they're unable to quit smoking.

The preventive approach to "silent" heart disease is fairly simple: Exercise! By walking thirty minutes five days per week or one hour three days per week, you reduce your chances of suffering a heart attack or dying of heart disease by 30-40%. Beyond that, exercise can serve as an early warning that there may be a heart problem.

So you see, even though we cannot prevent all heart disease, even against fixed risk factors you are not helpless. There is always something you can do to prevent heart disease.

But what if you've already suffered a heart attack or required an angioplasty, coronary stent, or bypass surgery? Does reducing your risk factors through diet and exercise help prevent a future problem? Yes. Absolutely!

So even if we can't prevent all heart disease, we can certainly prevent a great deal of it. The key is to not give up. Don't ever accept that a heart attack or bypass or angioplasty is inevitable. It isn't.

HEART DISEASE IN WOMEN

Sandra C is a 61-year-old bank manager with a ten-year history of high blood pressure and recently elevated cholesterol.

Question: **What is Sandra's risk for suffering a heart attack or stroke over the next ten years?**

Answer: 8%. In other words, Sandra has an 8% chance of a heart attack or stroke over the next decade. If she controls her hypertension and hypercholesterolemia and performs regular exercise, she may reduce her risk to below 1%.

Points to Remember:

- Heart disease kills 1 in 3 women, whereas breast cancer kills 1 in 31 women.

- Only 1 in 5 women think that heart disease is the biggest health risk.

- Heart disease may be "silent" in women.

- The three most common symptoms in women six months before they suffer a heart attack are fatigue, mild shortness of breath, and insomnia (difficulty sleeping).

How to Prevent Heart Disease

Think of the dozens of times over the years that your doctor has asked you to lose weight, lower your cholesterol, eat properly, and exercise regularly. Why haven't you followed through? Why haven't you made the effort?

It's because prevention isn't considered a priority. Prevention is "optional"—something that sounds good, and is hoped for, but is somewhat intangible. Prevention is something that "makes sense" but that you'll "get to later."

For example, if your sister surprised you by asking you to drive her to the hospital for her angioplasty procedure next Monday, would you be concerned? Of course you would. You'd be extremely worried. Angioplasty, although a common procedure, indicates that your sister has severe coronary artery disease. You wouldn't think twice about taking time off of work to be there.

What if, instead, your sister told you that her cholesterol was high and that her cardiologist wanted to prescribe medications that she wasn't in favor of taking? If she asked you to be present at her next doctor's appointment, would you cancel your golf game? Not likely.

Most people believe that if they have a coronary artery blockage, an angioplasty is more important than lowering their cholesterol. They could not be more wrong.

Not making cardiac prevention a priority is not your fault. Our healthcare system has to grant "prevention" the same status as any other "treatment." If so, then prevention becomes a treatment of heart disease.

SILENT HEART DISEASE IN DIABETES

David T: 59-year-old high school math teacher recently diagnosed with diabetes and a six-year history of high cholesterol. He has no complaints but is overweight and does not exercise. David knows that diabetes dramatically increases his risk for suffering a heart attack.

Question: **What is David's risk for suffering a heart attack or cardiac death over the next ten years?**

Answer: 15%. In other words, he has a 15% chance of a heart attack over the next decade.

If he controls his hypertension, hypercholesterolemia, and diabetes and performs regular exercise, he may reduce his risk to below 1%.

Points to Remember:

- Patients with diabetes have an 80-85% risk for developing cardiovascular disease

- 40% of people with diabetes may suffer a heart attack and not even know it (silent myocardial infarction).

How We Treat Heart Disease

I'd like to give a little background on how cardiologists approach heart disease. We do an excellent job of treating heart disease, but a poor job of preventing it. As physicians, we want to do a better job, but we are so busy treating heart disease that we don't have a lot of time to spend trying to prevent it. Since there is rarely enough time in our day to do both, we prioritize angioplasty and bypass surgery.

So, how do we treat heart disease? If you have heart disease—a blocked coronary artery—only three treatment options are available:

1. **Angioplasty**

2. **Bypass surgery**

3. **Medical management**

Angioplasty is a simple procedure in which the interventional cardiologist uses a small mesh stent placed on a balloon to prop open the blood vessel.

However, if the blockages are numerous or too complex for angioplasty, then your cardiologist will refer you to a surgeon for *bypass surgery*.

Many people with mild to moderate coronary artery stenosis (narrowing from blockages or plaque) may be followed medically rather than treated surgically. This is known as *medical management*. While medications do not shrink blockages (although there is evidence for coronary artery plaque regression with very low cholesterol levels), they can lower the risk factors that lead to a progression of heart disease.

The problem with angioplasty, bypass surgery, and even medical management is that these treatments are *reactive*—a response to a problem. Think of cardiac prevention as a new form of treating heart disease: a *proactive* option. Prevention is a proactive treatment that starts ten to twenty years before the others.

Determining Your Cardiac Risk

Be sure to schedule an appointment with your personal physician and have a complete evaluation performed. This is not only to make certain that it's safe for you to begin a diet and exercise program, but also to determine your risk of suffering a heart attack. Here's a little background on what your doctor does to assess your risk of a heart attack. For several decades, primary care physicians have relied on something known as a *Framingham risk score*. Don't worry too much about the terminology as it's not that important. Your calculated

Framingham risk score is basically your 10-year risk of suffering a heart attack or dying from one. All tests and treatments in cardiology are based upon this risk score.

Your *10-year risk* can be calculated either by hand or using an online risk calculator.

Note: In late 2013, new guidelines for cardiac prevention were published by the American Heart Association and American College of Cardiology representing a drastic departure from previous ones. In an attempt to simplify cardiac prevention, an online calculator is used to assess your 10-year risk of a heart attack. If your risk exceeds 7.5% (that is, 7.5% chance of having a heart attack or cardiac death within ten years) then you will be placed on a statin. These new guidelines have been met with some degree of controversy and will require modification, so I won't spend much time reviewing them here.

The bottom line is that patients are stratified into three groups based upon their Framingham risk scores: *low risk, intermediate risk,* and *high risk.* This risk score is based upon your age, gender, blood pressure, and cholesterol, among other things. Over the years, when it was found that the Framingham risk score may underestimate a person's true 10-year risk of suffering a heart attack, it was modified to include family history, type of cholesterol, and diabetes. Although a patient's calcium score has been found far more accurate in predicting future cardiac risk than the Framingham risk score, the latter has nevertheless played an important role in cardiac prevention.

Although you can calculate this score yourself with an online risk calculator, it's better to simply ask your doctor. If you have a Framingham risk score of 20%, you're considered high risk. In other words, you have a 20% chance of suffering a heart attack or dying of some form of heart disease over the next ten years. A low risk score is 1%.

If you think about it, the intermediate-risk patients (10% 10-year risk) should concern us the most, because a patient who has a low Framingham risk would be unlikely to have a cardiac problem, while a patient with high risk will be aggressively treated by a cardiologist focusing on prevention. Approximately a third of the U.S. population falls under the intermediate-risk category, yet these people are often undertreated or not treated at all!

Remember: The latest 2013 Cardiac Prevention Guidelines vary somewhat from the traditional Framingham Risk Assessment, so your doctor may use slightly different terminology and values for your risk assessment. Regardless, it's more important you understand the concept behind these risk calculators.

This book intended for two groups of people: those with numerous cardiac risk factors who have either an *intermediate* or a *high* Framingham risk score, and those who already have heart disease. Both groups should adopt a more aggressive approach to cardiac prevention by modifying their risk factors.

What is Your 10-Year Heart Disease Risk? (%)

Your doctor estimates your chances of having a heart attack or stroke over the next decade by using a simple online calculator.

www.cardiosource.org

To use this calculator you simply enter values for:

- **Gender:** Women tend to have cardiovascular disease later than men.

- **Age:** Age is our biggest risk factor. The older you are, the greater your likelihood of having severe heart disease.

- **Race:** Certain ethnicities have higher risk profiles than others.

- **Total Cholesterol**

- **HDL-Cholesterol:** Good cholesterol. Higher values are protective against cardiovascular disease.

- Systolic Blood Pressure

- **Treatment for High Blood Pressure:** Hypertension is closely associated with risk of heart attack and stroke.

- **Diabetes:** Diabetes shrinks your blood vessels and coats them with cholesterol plaque (hardening of the arteries).

- **Smoker:** The importance of stopping smoking can't be overemphasized.

Modifying Your Cardiac Risk Factors

Your primary care physician will take responsibility for controlling and monitoring your cardiac risk factors. Depending upon your risk factor profile, your doctor will recommend specific targets for your cholesterol, blood sugar, and blood pressure. Make sure you do all that you can to lower your risk factors for heart disease!

Lower Your Cholesterol

So many patients become confused when it comes to understanding their cholesterol that I recommend keeping it simple. Don't get bogged down in fancy terminology such as VAP panels, LDL subfractionation, apo A/B, myeloperoxidase, or VLDL. These terms are not necessary for your understanding. They're important, but just not for our purposes here. Instead, I'd like you to focus on your *LDL* or "bad" cholesterol, your *non-HDL cholesterol*, your *HDL cholesterol*, and your *triglycerides*. Rather than go through the biochemistry and physiology of cholesterol metabolism, I'll help you understand the important terms that you need to know. Also, don't become too concerned about the specific numeric values I mention regarding cholesterol, blood sugar, or even blood pressure. Over time, as you probably know, these targets change. What is important are the concepts behind why these values need to be low.

RISK FACTORS FOR HEART DISEASE (CORONARY-ARTERY DISEASE)

- Hypertension (high blood pressure)

- Hypercholesterolemia (high blood cholesterol)

- Diabetes

- Smoking

- Obesity

- Sedentary Lifestyle

- Family History

Source: Goff G, et al. 2013 ACC/AHA Guideline on the Assessment of Cardiovascular Risk: A Report of the American College of Cardiology/ American Heart Association Task Force on Practice Guidelines. *Circulation. 2013; published online before print November 12, 2013, doi:10.1161/01. cir.0000437741.48606.98*

LDL Cholesterol

When I use the term "cholesterol" I'm referring to LDL or "bad" cholesterol. What should your LDL level be?

If you have an intermediate risk factor for coronary artery disease but no documented heart disease (no previous heart attack, elevated calcium score, stent or angioplasty, stroke, or leg blockages), then your LDL target is below 100. However, I recommend that once you've brought your LDL below 100, you then use further dietary change to aim for an LDL below 70.

Note: Although the American Heart Association (AHA)'s 2013 Cardiac Prevention Guidelines have moved away from using LDL as the sole criterion for beginning a statin, I still recommend that LDL should be monitored routinely and used as a benchmark for cholesterol management.

If you have either coronary artery disease or diabetes, your LDL should be below 70. Once you've brought it below 70, I recommend that you modify your diet further to bring it below 60. This is because very low LDL levels have been linked to plaque regression, or shrinking of a soft cholesterol heart blockage. The units of cholesterol are not important (70 mg/dl). Just be sure to give your best effort to eat a diet low in saturated fat and cholesterol in order to keep your LDL below 70.

Also, did you notice that patients with diabetes are treated just as if they'd had a heart attack, stroke, by-pass surgery, or angioplasty? That's because people with diabetes have an extremely high incidence of cardiac events—on the order of 80-85%. We treat diabetic patients as if they have heart disease because it's so commonplace in that group.

The lower your LDL cholesterol, the lower will be your risk of heart disease. Conversely, the higher your LDL, the higher will be your risk of heart disease. Keeping it below 70, below 60 even, is what you should aim for. Once again, the 2013 AHA Cardiac Prevention Guidelines generated controversy because the authors concluded that a higher dosage of a cholesterol-reducing medication (a statin) is most responsible for lowering the risk of heart disease.

Non-HDL Cholesterol

Your non-HDL cholesterol should also be less than 100. Non-HDL cholesterol may be even more predictive of cardiac risk and can be calculated by taking your *total* cholesterol and subtracting the "good" or HDL cholesterol. This "non-good" or "everything bad" cholesterol includes all "bad" cholesterol particles. Typically, the non-HDL is around 30 points higher than the LDL cholesterol.

HDL and Triglycerides

What about your HDL and triglycerides? Exercise can improve or raise your HDL cholesterol. Although higher HDL levels can reduce your risk of heart disease, apart from exercise and niacin, it is difficult to raise the HDL. Your HDL should be above 40. For this reason, I would rather you focus on lowering your LDL than raising your HDL. Similarly, although important, I consider your triglyceride level to be a *secondary objective*. This is because your LDL and non-HDL levels are most closely associated with heart disease.

Triglycerides are a form of fat in your blood that helps store excess carbs and fat calories from your diet. Your triglyceride level should be less than 150.

Lower Your Blood Pressure

Your primary care physician will want your systolic blood pressure (top number reading) below 130. I advise patients to first ensure that their systolic pressure is less than 150 mm Hg. Once you've achieved this, work on getting your systolic blood pressure to be less than 140. There are two types of hypertension: *primary* and *secondary*. Most people have *primary hypertension*, meaning that they should first lose weight and decrease their intake of sodium, caffeine, and alcohol. *Secondary hypertension* is usually suspected when a patient is on four or even five medications at full dosages and still has poorly controlled blood pressure.

I would also suggest the purchase of a home blood pressure cuff for about fifty dollars at any drugstore. Measure your blood pressure twice a day for one week prior to your doctor's appointment and keep a written record for your doctor to review. I recommend taking one reading in the morning before medications and another at night before sleep. Your doctor will then use this information to adjust medications, if necessary.

Also, remember to bring all your medications to your appointments, along with your blood pressure cuff at least once for calibration. A fax machine is a convenient way of providing your doctor with your blood pressure trends when he or she adjusts your medications. Faxing your readings to your doctor can save you a lot of time and possibly save scheduling an office appointment.

Lower Your Blood Sugar

I consider diabetes to be the most dangerous risk factor for heart disease. When you have diabetes, your coronary arteries shrink and acquire a lining of cholesterol, reducing the success rate in case you need an angioplasty or bypass surgery. Therefore, over the long term you'll need to keep your blood sugar—hemoglobin A1c—below 6.0. Another reminder—if you have diabetes, I recommend that you consult with an endocrinologist and a nutritionist or dietician.

A Final Word about Prevention

Before we discuss diet and exercise, I want to reinforce the two important preventive concepts we have discussed so you can get the most out of this book. The first is to consider prevention to be a treatment of heart disease, no different than an angioplasty or bypass surgery. Second, take action to lower your risk factors. Don't just know what to do, go out and actually do what you know!

Prevention: The Most Important Treatment of Heart Disease

Over two decades as an interventional cardiologist (angioplasty specialist) I've treated many thousands of patients with heart disease. I've performed several thousand angiograms and angioplasty procedures and have recommended hundreds of patients for bypass surgery. Before their procedures, I've told all of my patients and their families, "Once you recover from your surgery the hard work will begin—preventing you from needing another one."

Describing prevention as a treatment is not a play on words. The most important treatment of any medical condition is to keep it from occurring in the first place. In order to do a better job at prevention, we—both patients and doctors—must completely change our approach to heart disease. We need to view prevention (lowering blood pressure, cholesterol, and blood sugar; losing weight through diet and exercise) as an actual treatment of heart disease, no different from medications, a heart bypass, or an angioplasty. In other words, controlling your blood pressure and lowering your cholesterol (prevention) is just as important as having an angioplasty (treatment). Losing weight and controlling your diabetes (prevention) is equally as important as a bypass surgery (treatment). Prevention *is* the most important treatment of heart disease.

WALKING 2 MILES PER DAY OR ANGIOPLASTY?

Walking 2 miles per day may reduce your risk of dying of heart disease by 30-40% or more.

People who can walk farther may have a 50-70% reduction in cardiac death.

Source: Kokkinos P. et al. Circulation. 2008; 117: 614-622
Source: Hakim AA. et al. N Engl J Med. 1998. Jan 8;338(2): 94-9

Doing What You Know Is More Important than Knowing What to Do

By now you're probably thinking, "I know this already. I know what to do. It's just that I haven't gotten around to doing it." The American Heart Association has spent tens of millions of dollars over the past several decades educating the public on the important of reducing cardiac risk factors (hypertension, smoking, diabetes, hypercholesterolemia), performing regular exercise, and eating a healthy diet. So just about everyone knows the importance of modifying your cardiac risk factors. But when it comes to preventing heart disease and making lifestyle changes, knowing what to do is never the problem. It's doing what you already know!

Everyone knows smoking is bad for you, right? Did you know that more than 20% of men and women still smoke?

Everyone knows that exercise is good for you, but were you aware that nearly one-third of all Americans don't exercise at all?

Everyone knows that being overweight is unhealthy, yet nearly 70% of Americans are overweight!

We all know that high cholesterol will lead to heart disease, yet more than forty million Americans have elevated cholesterol.

Everyone also knows that high blood pressure is the "silent killer." Still, one-third of Americans have hypertension, and more than half of those do not have their blood pressure under control.

Why don't we just make changes in our lifestyle? Why can't we follow through? We procrastinate about prevention because it's not considered a priority. Eating more healthy or getting regular exercise is something that you get to—later . Contrast this to if you were told you needed a bypass surgery. Would you put that off until next year? Of course not. Our system prioritizes procedures. So does your doctor, and so do you. We must prioritize prevention.

Benefits of Exercise on Heart Health

1. Weight loss

2. Improves blood pressure

3. Reduces bad (LDL) cholesterol

4. Improves good (HDL) cholesterol

5. Improves diabetes

6. Reduces risk of certain types of cancer: breast cancer, colon cancer, endometrial cancer.

7. Strengthens bones and muscles.

Source; Meyers J. Circulation. **2003;** 107: **e2-e5**

PART TWO:

USING DIET AND EXERCISE TO PREVENT HEART DISEASE

The Best Exercise Program and the Best Diet Program

By now, I hope I've convinced you that you can do a lot more to reduce your chances of developing heart disease. Cardiac prevention is a realistic and tangible goal, but it does require you to make lowering your risk factors through weight loss, diet, and exercise a daily priority. This takes commitment and discipline.

But how do you actually do this? Where do you begin? Which diet should you follow? What exercise program is best?

Although this may seem overwhelming, it's actually pretty easy.

In case you're wondering why I don't have my own diet or exercise program for you to follow, it's because I believe the last thing the world needs right now is another fad diet. The second-to-last thing the world needs is another exercise program.

My patients often ask me, "What is the best diet?"

and "Should I join a fitness center?" My answer is simple. The best diet program is the one you'll be on five years from now. The same applies to your exercise program. Don't get caught up in "miracle" weight-loss diets or rigorous "body-transforming" exercise programs. Although it is true that a more stringent diet and a more rigorous exercise program will help you lose weight faster, it's unrealistic to think you will stick to them for very long.

For example, have you tried a low-carb diet? Of course you have. It was a huge fad a decade or more ago. It still is. It works! If you don't eat carbs, you'll lose weight (mostly because you're eating less calories!). The problem is that not many other foods are left if you cut out an entire food group, so it's not a good long-term strategy.

The same goes for your exercise program. There are so many excellent high-impact aerobic programs available from late-night TV infomercials. These do a fantastic job of getting you in shape over a few months. But not everyone has the dedication or the ability to follow them for long periods of time. They're not easy; that's why they work! Do you really think you'll be able to continue this type of exercise program five years from now?

If you pick diets and exercise programs you know you can't keep up with, you'll become frustrated.

Weight Loss as Prevention

Weight loss is the single most important step that *you* can take to prevent heart disease. Losing weight improves your blood sugar, blood pressure, and cholesterol and even reduces your risk for cancer. Yet most people who are on a diet simply want to look better.

With so many diets and exercise programs available, you'd think no one would be overweight. We should be a country of supermodels. Yet when you visit your local mall or beach, nearly 70% of the people you see are either obese or overweight. Also, nearly half of us are on a diet at any one time. That means most of your friends, family, neighbors, and co-workers are dieting. So if everyone is dieting and exercising, why are so many people overweight?

The problem is that diets help you lose weight but aren't very effective at helping you maintain the reduced weight. In fact, as you've most likely experienced, the faster you lose weight, the higher the likelihood that you'll gain it all back. So when it comes to dieting, your goal should be weight loss *followed by maintenance of that healthier weight.*

For the rest of this book, I'd like to share a few concepts and strategies about dieting to help you keep from regaining the weight that you work so hard to lose.

Choosing the Best Diet for You

Choosing a diet isn't that hard. I don't recommend that you spend a lot of time deciding which diet to follow. Pick a plan that interests you and start following it.

What's the best diet? The best diet is the one you can live with. Stick with proven programs such as Weight Watchers®, Nutrisystem®, or Jenny Craig®, just to name a few. Fortunately there are dozens of different diets to choose from, so you'll have no trouble finding one that fits your tastes, lifestyle, and personality. Since all diets will help you lose weight, it really doesn't matter which one you pick, so don't waste a lot of time deciding. This is because the real 'work' will be to avoid regaining the weight you lost through dieting. So find a program you like and get started.

You may be wondering why I recommend that you choose a name-brand diet instead of creating my own diet for you. It's because such programs as Weight

Watchers®, Nutrisystem®, or Jenny Craig® have a proven track record of success. They have expertly developed meal plans to satisfy your hunger and use sophisticated advertising techniques to keep you motivated. Honestly, I could not possibly create a better program than these. As I have said before, the last thing that the world needs is another diet and more important than losing weight is maintaining your weight loss. So choose one of the most popular plans and follow it!

Long-Term Success vs. Short-Term Gains

Remember to have realistic expectations with any diet plan that you choose. The success of a diet should be judged over the course of many years, not weeks or months. I recommend that you lose no more than two to four pounds per month. You may not be too happy with such a patient approach, but the faster you lose weight, the more likely it is that you'll regain it all back. If you've put on twenty pounds over the past two years you shouldn't expect to lose this over three months.

Also, avoid a diet that cuts the amount of calories you eat too aggressively. Overly restrictive diets will shock your system and be too difficult to follow. It's not a good long-term strategy.

One Size Does Not Fit All

Each person's weight loss goals, medical history, physiology, metabolism, genetics, lifestyle, and preferences are obviously different. When you evaluate a diet, make sure that it fits your personal goals and lifestyle. Also be aware that your weight-loss and fitness goals will change over time. They are not static. The nutrition and fitness goals you have at age 40 will be much different when you are 60 years old. Your diet must adapt to these changes.

Exercise as Prevention

Walk, Don't Run: The Benefits of Walking

Your exercise program will consist of walking on flat ground at a conversational pace, for no more than thirty minutes, five days a week. That's all. I don't recommend a lot of fancy equipment, technology, or gym memberships. If you can afford the latest treadmill, techno gadgets, and personal trainers, then be my guest. A comfortable pair of walking shoes is really all you'll need.

No jogging, running, jumping up and down, race-walking, or hill-climbing. There's certainly nothing wrong with jogging or these other aerobic activities, but you'll just end up either suffering an injury or avoiding your exercise altogether. Just go for a leisurely walk on flat ground, thirty minutes, five days a week. Do this and you'll reduce your chances of dying from a heart attack by 30-40% or more. Walking is more effective at preventing heart disease than a cardiac stent!

In addition, a walking program will help you develop small blood vessels known as *collaterals*. Collateral vessels can serve to bypass blockages in your coronary arteries. If you think of your major coronary arteries as freeways, collaterals are like surface streets. Should you suffer a heart attack, these collaterals can be life-saving.

You're not limited to walking outdoors, either. You may swim, use a treadmill, stair-stepper, elliptical machine, or exercise bike. What you exercise with doesn't make a difference. Just perform low-intensity aerobic exercise for a sufficient period of time and do it regularly.

Exercise also improves your "good" cholesterol, or HDL, and as I pointed out earlier, people with higher HDL are better protected against heart disease.

Overdoing It

If thirty minutes of exercise is good, then an hour would be better, right? If walking is good, then running should be better, right?

It is true that the more you exercise the better it is, and ultimately I would like you to walk for one hour five days per week, but that's too much too soon. Just stick with your thirty-minute program for now. If you overdo your exercise program, not only will you injure yourself, you'll also burn out. No one wants to perform rigorous exercise. That's why, for high-intensity work-outs, most people need a class, a personal trainer, or a video. You can't do them on your own, at least not for long. It's too difficult to stay motivated.

The point is not to worry about intensity or heart rate. You don't even have to perspire. You just want to walk at the pace of a leisurely stroll. You shouldn't be breathless.

After two to three months your exercise program will become a part of your routine. As you become more advanced, you may then increase your exercise time to forty-five minutes and eventually to an hour. However, it's not required.

You're probably thinking that a thirty-minute walk on a treadmill is way too easy to be effective. It's actually a lot harder than you think. Don't forget that you're walking five days a week, not just when you remember to or feel like it. It'll take a lot of self-discipline. The key is consistency. It is *consistent* exercise that allows you to maintain your weight loss.

Of course, walking is not as effective for burning calories as running or jumping. But remember, our goal is for you to maintain your weight loss. There's no purpose in trying to lose a lot of weight rapidly with an aggressive diet and exercise program but being unable to realistically follow through with either, then regain-ing your weight. Again, if you injure yourself by over-aggressive exercise, you'll sabotage both your exercise program and your diet.

In summary, just go for a leisurely walk for thirty

minutes on flat ground at a conversational pace most days of the week and you'll do just fine!

One Final Reminder: Small Changes, Simple Changes

Now that you've chosen your diet and a new exercise program, I'd like to once again emphasize the importance of being patient.

When it comes to losing weight, don't be overenthusiastic. Go slow. Avoid doing too much too fast. If you make drastic changes to your diet and exercise program you'll surely burn out and get discouraged.

No matter what diet plan you follow, be sure to take the most conservative weight loss route. In other words, if you can lose ten pounds in a month on a more aggressive program, choose a path where you only lose two pounds in a month. I know what you're thinking: "Two pounds a month? Forget it! I want to lose two pounds a week!" But if you lose weight too quickly, even though it's possible, severe changes to your diet and exercise will be required. You don't want this. You need to lose weight gradually, almost imperceptibly. Gradual weight loss becomes permanent weight loss. Small and simple changes to your diet and exercise over the course of a year will become permanent lifestyle changes.

So no matter what diet program you're on, and regardless of the stated time frame for weight loss, I suggest you extend this to expectation to twelve months.

When it comes to your exercise, once again, I recommend that you not exceed thirty minutes five days a week for at least a month. I can't say it often enough: If you're overaggressive, you'll burn out.

How to Improve Any Diet

Losing weight is easy. Keeping it off is difficult. Do you remember the last time you went on a diet and lost ten pounds? How did you do it?

Every diet is effective at helping you lose weight initially. You avoided certain foods and limited the number of calories you ate. You also probably started an exercise program to help increase your metabolism. It worked! You were pleased with the scale readings and the way you looked in the mirror. Your clothes began to fit better. Losing that first ten pounds wasn't so hard!

Maintaining your weight loss is what's really difficult. You see, it's easy to be enthusiastic about starting a new diet. You're willing to invest a lot of time and energy buying the proper foods, exercising, and planning meals. Over time, however, your enthusiasm begins to fade as the novelty of the diet wears off. Sticking to your diet became a daily struggle. The pounds don't seem to come off as easily as before. You have less energy. You're always hungry, and you start craving the foods you're no longer supposed to eat. After a while, you begin to question whether the effort is even worth it. With your busy schedule and the pressures of everyday life, it becomes increasingly difficult to find the time to stick to your program. Eventually, you revert to your original eating patterns, stop exercising, and regain the weight you spent so much time and effort trying to lose. It becomes frustrating and demoralizing.

What happened? Why is losing weight so easy, yet keeping it off so difficult?

The only way to maintain your weight is to balance the number of calories you eat against the number you burn off. Because there's no way to measure how many calories you burn, even if you count calories in your diet, you won't know how much to eat. As a result, you're constantly dieting. You lose weight, gain it back, then try to lose weight again. Another fad diet makes the headlines, and you start this cycle all over again. In the end, you really haven't lost weight, because whatever weight you lost, you regained. I call this cycle of dieting "the weight-loss yo-yo." What you lose today, you'll be sure to gain back later.

Two Ways to Help You Maintain
Your Weight Loss

So how do you keep from regaining the weight that you worked so hard to lose? I would like you to consider incorporating *two simple strategies* that can help your diet program more effectively maintain your weight. This common-sense approach is unproven, so you'll have to decide if it works for you or not. I really hope that it does. The proven alternatives, which your doctor may recommend, are medications and gastric bypass surgery.

First, you need to *determine your calorie equilibrium*. In other words, you need to be able to estimate how much to eat each day. If you eat more calories than you burn, you'll gain weight.

Second, you need to achieve *satiety*. No diet will work if you're always hungry. And what are you typically hungry for? Junk food! That's why you also have to *curb your craving* for junk food. If you feel cheated that you have to avoid certain foods, you're more likely to binge or even abandon your diet altogether.

1. Determining Your Calorie Equilibrium: Estimating How Much to Eat Each Day

When you hear the word "calorie," mostly because of highly effective advertising of products like diet soda, the first thought that probably comes to mind is "bad." When it comes to dieting, most people think that zero calories are "good," and the more calories a food contains, the worse it is. It's not true. A calorie is simply a measure of the energy a food contains. A calorie is neither good nor bad.

If you eat more calories than you burn, this excess energy will be stored as fat, and you'll gain weight. We call this *positive calorie balance.*

In order to lose weight, you simply have to take in fewer calories than you burn. This is known as *negative calorie balance.*

To maintain your weight, you need to reach a *calorie balance equilibrium.* In this case, you're eating the same amount of calories that you expend.

When you start a new diet, it's easy to be in a *negative calorie balance*, because you have simply cut back on how many calories you are eating. This is why you lose weight initially. Most of the weight you lose is probably water and not actually fat. But that doesn't matter, because the psychological benefit of losing weight is what you're after. But because dieting slows your metabolism, you'll need exercise to counter this. You gain the weight back because your calorie equilibrium varies depending on what and how much you eat, and your activities.

Although there isn't a way to know precisely what this equilibrium is on a given day, there is a way to estimate it.

Let's use a simple analogy. Nowadays all cars have a miles-per-gallon (MPG) gauge that calculates your *instantaneous* and *average* MPG use. If you have a lead foot and do a lot of jack-rabbit starts, your instantaneous mileage could be ten MPG. Five minutes later, cruising on the freeway with your foot lightly on the accelerator you may be getting thirty-five MPG. In reality, the instantaneous MPG reading is pretty useless. What *is* useful is the *average* miles-per-gallon.

It's the same with your calorie equilibrium. It's impossible to know how many calories you should eat on a given day, because it varies with your activity. That's like estimating your weekly MPG on the basis of one instantaneous MPG reading. You can't!

The only reason to care about your car's average MPG is to save money at the gas pump. Similarly, the only reason to estimate your calorie equilibrium is to maintain or lose weight.

Let's say you want to spend seventy dollars a week on gas. Because gas prices change, as does the distance you drive, the only variable you have significant control over is *how you drive*. To get more mileage from the same amount of gas you have to modify your *driving behavior*.

What happens if the MPG gauge in your car is broken? How will you know whether or not your driving behavior will allow you to keep your gasoline bill at seventy dollars for the week? The only way to know will be your bill at the pump at week's end. If your gas bill is ninety dollars for the week, then you'll need to change your driving behavior. If it's still seventy dollars, you can continue driving in the same manner, driving approximately the same distance, and using gas stations with similar prices.

If you think of this in terms of diet and exercise, your *body weight* at the end of each week represents your *gas bill* at the pump. The number of calories in the foods you eat varies, as does the price of gas. Your exercise, or lack of it, compares to the distance you drive. Your eating behavior is like your driving behavior. It's not an exact parallel, but you get the idea. So if your weight at the end of the week is nearly the same as it was at the end of last week, then you have achieved your *calorie-balance equilibrium.* On the other hand, if you wanted to continue losing weight, you'd have to change your eating habits, your exercise, or both.

In summary, you can get a pretty good estimate of how much food to eat on any given day by weighing yourself at the end of the week. All you have to do to maintain your weight is to:

a. **Perform consistent exercise.** (drive the same distance each day)

b. **Eat consistently.** Don't add or skip meals. (your driving habits)

c. **Monitor your weight at the end of each week.** (your gas bill at the pump)

It's easy to understand the principle of exercising every day and weighing yourself once per week, but how do you eat consistently? The specific diet program that you're on will outline how many meals and snacks you are allowed each day. For example, I advocate three meals and five snacks per day. Of course, you'll also want to include a few cheat meals or snacks, too! Whether you're hungry or not, you eat three meals and five snacks per day. This regulates how much you eat and when. If you've gained two pounds at the end of the week, you'll need to increase your exercise, cut back on your snacks, or both. This is just a simple example, but you get the idea!

2. Satiety: Curbing Your Appetite

You can't maintain your weight loss if you're always hungry. You have to be satisfied with the meals that your diet plan provides. Whether or not you're satiated after a meal depends upon two factors: the *amount* of food you eat and the *types* of foods you eat. Of the two, I believe it is the *types* of foods that you eat that plays a bigger role in suppressing your appetite.

Let's assume you've just eaten dinner. You enjoyed a nice salad with vinaigrette and a main course of cheese pasta with broiled chicken breast. For dessert you had a frozen yogurt with some fresh fruit. The serving sizes were generous, and you didn't feel you were being restricted.

But here's the problem. You're still hungry! Why?

It's not just because you've reduced the *amount* of food you're eating. Although it is true you'll have to reduce your calorie intake, that's not the real reason you're still hungry. It's the *type* of food you're eating, or avoiding, that determines satiety. For instance, if you're in the mood for pepperoni pizza and have to settle for broiled salmon, no matter how much salmon you eat you'll still be craving pizza.

You've developed preferences for eating, over several decades, that I to refer to as your *eating behavior*. You know *what* you like to eat, *why* you like to eat, *when* you like to eat, and *how much* you like to eat. You've adopted a set of likes and dislikes that are part of who you are. When you have to change your *eating behavior* through dieting, even though you have more than enough food to eat, you'll feel cheated. Also, after a lifetime growing to love certain foods, such as junk food, suddenly cutting them out will make you crave them even more. This leads to frustration, and you might end up bingeing on the very foods you're trying to avoid, or even quit your diet completely.

The problem is compounded if you've had a very unhealthy diet over the years. If so, you'll have to make a lot of changes to correct your eating behavior. This is going to take a long time. Changing your diet is as difficult as changing the hand you write with. If you're right-handed and are asked to only write with your left hand starting tomorrow, your first reaction will be to think it's impossible. You'll quickly become frustrated and probably quit trying. But what if you're given one year to make the change? You could do it!

With any diet, you also have to avoid certain "problem" or junk foods and find acceptable substitutes. Unfortunately, these are usually the foods that you crave the most. You'll want to limit foods high in simple carbs, saturated fats, sugar, sodium, and cholesterol. It's not that you can never enjoy a cheeseburger and fries or chocolate cake and ice cream ever again, because these could be part of your occasional cheat meals, but for the most part it's better to find healthy alternatives.

In order to suppress your cravings for junk foods, you'll need to substitute healthier foods with the same general characteristics. So if you're in the mood for a large serving of chocolate ice cream, an apple won't satisfy that craving. For ice cream, you may want to substitute a yogurt parfait, a smoothie, or frozen yogurt.

It's important both to understand the characteristics of the foods we crave and what factors make a meal satisfying.

The Physiology and Psychology of Eating: Curbing Hunger

Several factors make a meal satisfying. Taste, texture, aroma, and other sensations associated with eating contribute to our feelings of satiety. Sharing a meal with friends and family can also be enjoyable and relaxing.

In describing how your body works we use the term "physiology." Your body's physiologic responses to eating are predictable. Following a meal, blood flow increases to your stomach and intestines to aid in the digestion of food. As your metabolism increases, chemicals released in your digestive system signal various areas of your brain.

In order to feel satiated after eating, you must experience the physical actions of chewing, tasting, and swallowing, as well as abdominal distension. That's why, if you're hungry and try to curb your appetite by chewing a piece of gum, it doesn't work. Similarly, a supersized diet cola may distend your abdomen and satisfy your sweet tooth, but you'll still be hungry. When you're really hungry, small portions from a tasting menu won't satisfy you and will only increase your appetite.

In addition to your body's physical response to a meal, eating is also associated with many *psychological* responses. Certain tastes and smells have powerful associations from our past experiences. For example, chocolate-chip cookies may bring back enjoyable memories from your childhood.

A pleasant meal can be a welcome reward to a long, stressful day of work. Many people, too busy to eat breakfast or lunch, are famished by the end of the day and look forward to a long, relaxing dinner with family and friends as the perfect reward. This is why overly restrictive diets fail. Eating is a pleasurable experience.

It's enjoyable and comforting both physiologically and psychologically. Rather than deny yourself the pleasure of a satisfying meal, I suggest creating meal plans that give you the enjoyable and satisfying experience you deserve!

Finally, you are aware of eating disorders and other psychological conditions such as overeating in response to anxiety, depression, or anger. These serious disorders require the attention of mental-health professionals.

The Seven Characteristics of a Satisfying Meal

With this understanding of how our bodies and minds play a role in our feeling of satiety, how can we create meals to suppress our appetite and cravings?

I believe *seven food characteristics* are required to make a meal satisfying. If any of these seven is missing, you'll still be hungry even if the quantity of food is sufficient.

It's not necessary to find foods that meet all of these seven characteristics, but you'll need to create meals which do. In other words, when preparing any meal, be sure to select foods that meet the following criteria:

1. Taste—sweet, salty, fatty, sour, spicy?
2. Texture—crunchy, creamy, chewy, gooey, fizzy?
3. Temperature—good hot or good cold?
4. Aroma—pleasing aroma?

5. Satiety—cause abdominal distention, make you feel full?

6. Sensation—require chewing, pleasant to swallow?

7. Social setting—consumed in pleasant and relaxing circumstances?

SEVEN CHARACTERISTICS OF A SATISFYING MEAL	
Taste	1. Taste—sweet, salty, fatty, sour, spicy?
Texture	2. Texture—crunchy, creamy, chewy, gooey, fizzy?
Temperature	3. Temperature—good hot or good cold?
Aroma	4. Aroma—pleasing aroma?
Satiety	5. Satiety—cause abdominal distention, make you feel full?
Sensation	6. Sensation—require chewing, pleasant to swallow?
Social	7. Social Setting—consumed in pleasant and relaxing circumstances?

Now consider our previous example in terms of pizza. If piping-hot pepperoni pizza is what you're craving during Monday night football but your diet plan calls for broiled salmon and broccoli, it's not going to work. No amount of salmon will satisfy your hunger for pizza. Salmon, as a stand-alone food, does not fulfill the seven criteria. Even if you're allowed as much salmon as you want, you'll still be hungry for pizza.

In order to satisfy your pizza craving, you'll have

	THE 7 SATISFYING CHARACTERISTICS OF SALMON	THE 7 SATISFYING CHARACTERISTICS OF PIZZA
Taste	X	X
Texture	X	X
Temperature	X	X
Aroma		X
Satiety		X
Sensation		X
Social		X

to find a substitute with all or most of pizza's seven food characteristics. How about spaghetti? Will your craving for pizza be satisfied by spaghetti smothered with tomato sauce and mozzarella cheese, plus a side order of garlic bread? Let's say you went to your local pizzeria and ordered your favorite combination, only to be told that the pizza oven broke just before your pie was ready. What would you do? Would you accept the complimentary spaghetti, or would you walk out?

You might not be happy at first, but chances are you'd probably settle for the spaghetti. After the meal, would you be satisfied, or would you go to another pizzeria and get a pizza to go? Your appetite would be satisfied, because spaghetti has many of the seven characteristics of a satisfying meal as pizza.

But since spaghetti smothered with cheese and garlic bread bathed in butter is not much healthier than pepperoni pizza, we have to find alternatives. How about nonfat American cheese instead of mozzarella? What about replacing the butter on your garlic bread with pesto? You'd probably consider that an acceptable substitute.

The 7 Satisfying Characteristics of Pizza	Spaghetti with Non-fat American Cheese
Taste	X	X
Texture	X	X
Temperature	X	X
Aroma	X	X
Satiety	X	X
Sensation	X	X
Social	X	X

Food Substitutions vs. Complete Meals

Given the previous discussion, you might anticipate several chapters of food substitutions. For example, we could analyze the characteristics of the most common food cravings and find substitutions for chocolate cake, ice cream, pastries, or potato chips. But this would be too complicated and time consuming. Remember, successful diet programs are simple, easy to follow, and don't require too much time for meal planning.

Rather than fret over individual food alternatives, try instead to create meals from foods your diet allows that will also fulfill the seven food characteristics. So if you didn't want to cook spaghetti but had the craving for pizza, you could create an entire meal that meets our seven criteria.

In other words, even though you craved pizza, you could still leave the table satisfied because your meal met all of the seven characteristics. The point is that you can see how easy and quick it can be to create meals using foods allowed on your diet program that leave you satisfied throughout the day! It's not only easy, it's fun to do!

If you're following Weight Watchers®, Nutrisystem®, or Jenny Craig® just be sure that each meal you create satisfies most or all seven essential characteristics. If you're allowed to choose your foods, pick them for the same reason.

Regardless of how hungry you are, the following menus are examples of the types of foods that could

THE 7 SATISFYING CHARACTERISTICS	TASTE	TEXT	TEMP	AROMA	SATIETY	SENS	SOCIAL
Pizza	X	X	X	X	X	X	X
Soup: Chicken Noodle or Vegetable	X	X	X		X	X	
Carbonated Water with Lemon	X	X	X		X		
Coffee or Tea	X		X	X		X	X
Tuna Melt	X	X	X	X	X	X	

suppress your appetite for breakfast, lunch, and dinner. This is not intended to be a comprehensive meal plan but only an illustration of how to create meals with the seven satisfying food characteristics.

In summary, although it's possible to analyze and find substitutes for particular foods, it's best to create meals that include all seven satisfying characteristics (taste, texture, temperature, aroma, satiety, sensation, social setting). If you do, there's a good chance that you'll leave the table feeling satisfied after every meal.

Breakfast Choice Examples

	TASTE	TEXT	TEMP	AROMA	SATIETY	SENS	SOCIAL
Coffee or Tea	TASTE		TEMP				SOCIAL
French Toast	TASTE	TEXT	TEMP	AROMA	SATIETY	SENS	
Milk	TASTE				SATIETY	SENS	
Juice	TASTE		TEMP		SATIETY	SENS	
Fruit: Strawberries, Cantaloupe, Honeydew Melon	TASTE	TEXT					
Pancakes	TASTE	TEXT	TEMP	AROMA	SATIETY	SENS	SOCIAL
Canadian Bacon	TASTE	TEXT		AROMA	SATIETY	SENS	
Apple Cinnamon Oat-meal	TASTE	TEXT	TEMP	AROMA	SATIETY	SENS	SOCIAL
Granola	TASTE	TEXT				SENS	
Blueberry Muffins	TASTE	TEXT	TEMP	AROMA	SATIETY	SENS	SOCIAL

LUNCH CHOICE EXAMPLES	TASTE	TEXT	TEMP	AROMA	SATIETY	SENS	SOCIAL
Carbonated Water with Lemon	TASTE	TEXT	TEMP		SATIETY		
Coffee or Tea	TASTE		TEMP	AROMA			SOCIAL
Yogurt Smoothie	TASTE	TEXT	TEMP		SATIETY	SENS	
Chicken Quesadilla	TASTE	TEXT	TEMP	AROMA	SATIETY	SENS	SOCIAL
Meatball Parmesan	TASTE	TEXT	TEMP	AROMA	SATIETY	SENS	SOCIAL
Tuna Melt	TASTE	TEXT	TEMP		SATIETY	SENS	
Chicken Salad	TASTE	TEXT			SATIETY	SENS	
Soup: Chicken Noodle or Vegetable	TASTE	TEXT	TEMP		SATIETY	SENS	SOCIAL
Pasta Salad	TASTE	TEXT			SATIETY	SENS	

DINNER CHOICE EXAMPLES

	TASTE	TEXT	TEMP	AROMA	SATIETY	SENS	SOCIAL
Carbonated Water with Lemon	TASTE	TEXT	TEMP	AROMA	SATIETY		
Coffee or Tea	TASTE		TEMP	AROMA		SENS	SOCIAL
Chicken Wrap	TASTE	TEXT	TEMP	AROMA	SATIETY	SENS	SOCIAL
Salad with Vinaigrette	TASTE	TEXT			SATIETY	SENS	
Spaghetti	TASTE	TEXT	TEMP	AROMA	SATIETY	SENS	SOCIAL
Cheese Ravioli	TASTE	TEXT	TEMP	AROMA	SATIETY	SENS	
Lasagna	TASTE	TEXT	TEMP	AROMA	SATIETY	SENS	SOCIAL
Meatloaf and Mashed Potatoes	TASTE	TEXT	TEMP	AROMA	SATIETY	SENS	SOCIAL
Cheese Pasta with Chicken	TASTE	TEXT		AROMA	SATIETY	SENS	SOCIAL
Italian Herb Flatbread Pizza	TASTE	TEXT	TEMP	AROMA	SATIETY	SENS	SOCIAL

Putting It All Together

Thank you for allowing me to share my philosophy of cardiac prevention with you. I hope this book has been of value to you and given you encouragement and motivation.

I truly believe we can do a much better job of preventing heart disease through simple lifestyle changes. It's what we've known all along. Do your best to control your blood pressure, blood sugar, and cholesterol, stop smoking, eat a healthy diet, and exercise regularly.

For nearly two decades my patients have asked me what the best diet is. Dieting to lose weight is necessary, but it's not the total solution. Maintaining your post-diet weight is what's difficult but essential. I hope my strategies of weight maintenance will work for you, and I wish you the best of luck in staying healthy so that you can avoid needing my services or that of any of my 50,000 cardiology colleagues!

About the Author

Dr. Gregg Yamada has been a practicing cardiologist in Honolulu for nearly two decades. Despite his background as an angioplasty specialist, Dr. Yamada believes that many cardiac procedures could be avoided if lifestyle changes are adopted early on. Despite having been board certified in nuclear cardiology, cardiovascular CT imaging, interventional (angioplasty) cardiology, cardiovascular disease and internal medicine, Dr. Yamada considers himself more of a general cardiologist. His focus is to help his patients do their best to prevent heart disease.

33669235R00058

Made in the USA
San Bernardino, CA
07 May 2016